How Iodine Shapes Your Thyroid

Vital Insights and Essential Knowledge

By

Calvin M. Duncan

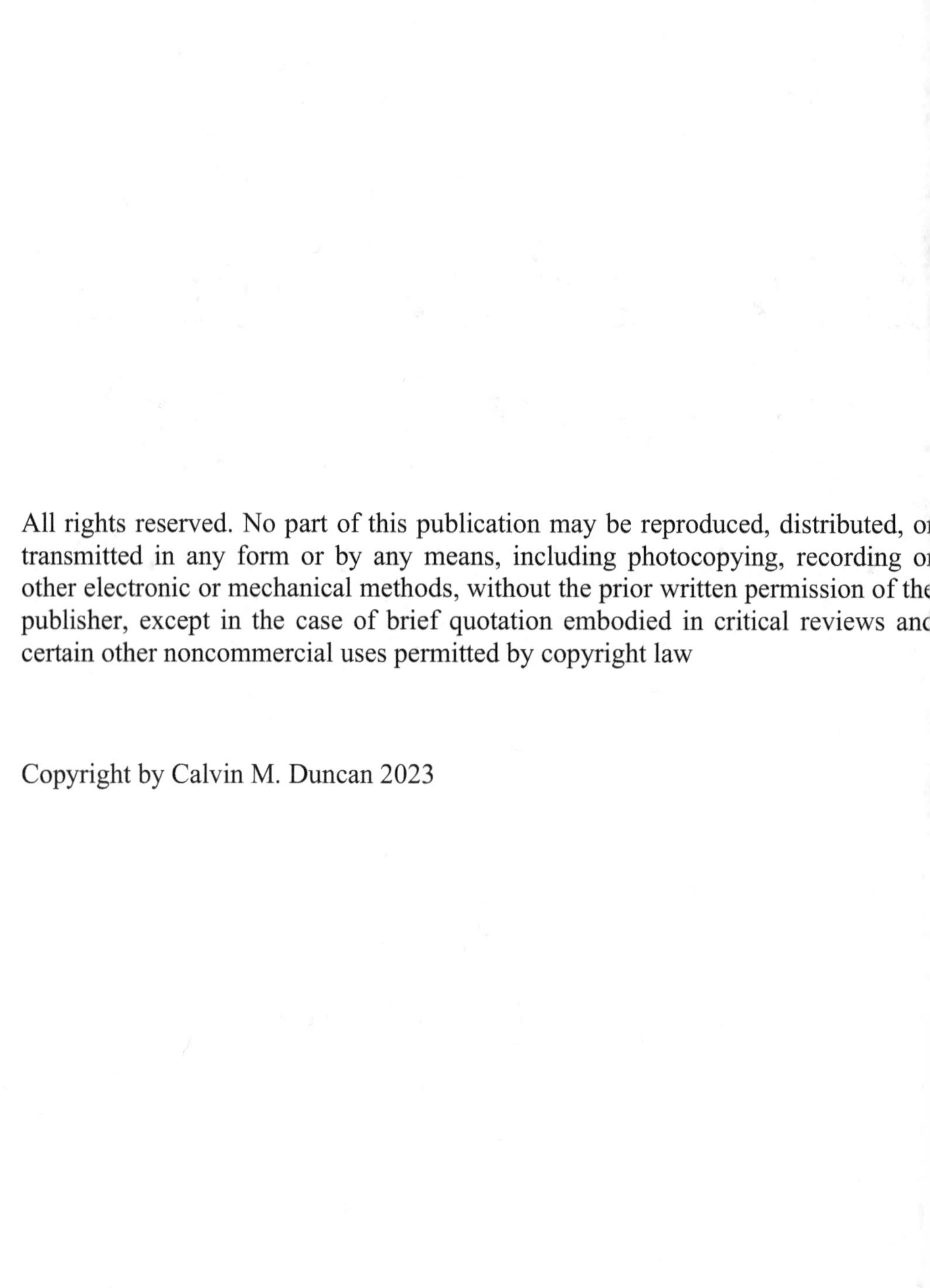

All rights reserved. No part of this publication may be reproduced, distributed, or transmitted in any form or by any means, including photocopying, recording or other electronic or mechanical methods, without the prior written permission of the publisher, except in the case of brief quotation embodied in critical reviews and certain other noncommercial uses permitted by copyright law

Copyright by Calvin M. Duncan 2023

TABLE OF CONTENTS

INTRODUCTION

Understanding The Thyroid Gland

The thyroid gland is a small, butterfly-shaped organ located in the neck, just below the Adam's apple. Despite its size, the thyroid plays a crucial role in regulating various bodily functions and maintaining overall health. In this section, we will delve into understanding the thyroid gland, its anatomy, functions, and significance in the human body.

The thyroid gland consists of two lobes connected by a thin bridge of tissue called the isthmus. Each lobe is roughly the size of a walnut and is composed of millions of tiny, specialized cells known as thyroid follicles. These follicles are responsible for producing and storing thyroid hormones.

The thyroid gland's primary function is to synthesize and release two essential hormones: thyroxine (T4) and triiodothyronine (T3). These hormones are iodine-based and play a vital role in regulating the body's metabolism, which is the process by which the body converts food into energy.

T4 is the more abundant thyroid hormone produced by the thyroid gland. It is relatively inactive on its own but serves as a precursor to T3. T3 is the more biologically active hormone and is responsible for controlling metabolic processes throughout the body.

Regulation of Thyroid Function

The release of thyroid hormones is controlled by a feedback mechanism involving the hypothalamus and the pituitary gland. When the body's cells need more thyroid hormones, the hypothalamus releases thyrotropin-releasing hormone (TRH). TRH signals the pituitary gland to produce and release thyroid-stimulating hormone (TSH). TSH, in turn, stimulates the thyroid gland to produce and release T4 and T3.

This feedback loop ensures that the body's metabolic rate remains stable and that there are adequate thyroid hormones circulating in the bloodstream to meet the body's demands.

Thyroid Hormones and Metabolism

Thyroid hormones have a profound impact on metabolism. They influence how the body uses energy, the rate at which it burns calories, and the production of heat. When thyroid hormone

levels are too low (a condition known as hypothyroidism), the body's metabolic processes slow down, leading to symptoms like fatigue, weight gain, and cold intolerance. Conversely, when thyroid hormone levels are too high (a condition known as hyperthyroidism), the body's metabolic processes become overactive, resulting in symptoms such as weight loss, anxiety, and heat intolerance.

Other Functions of the Thyroid Gland

Beyond its role in metabolism, the thyroid gland also plays a crucial part in various other bodily functions. It influences the cardiovascular system by affecting heart rate and blood pressure. Additionally, it impacts the digestive system, helping to regulate bowel movements. Thyroid hormones are essential for the development and growth of tissues in children and the maintenance of healthy bones and muscles in adults.

Thyroid Health and Disorders

Maintaining the health of the thyroid gland is vital for overall well-being. Thyroid disorders are common and can lead to a range of health issues. Hypothyroidism, characterized by low thyroid hormone levels, can cause fatigue, weight gain, depression, and cognitive impairment. Hyperthyroidism, characterized by high thyroid hormone levels, can result in anxiety, weight loss, and heart palpitations.

Autoimmune conditions like Hashimoto's thyroiditis and Graves' disease can affect the thyroid gland, leading to chronic thyroid problems. Thyroid nodules, which are lumps or growths on the thyroid, are also common and may be benign or malignant.

In conclusion, the thyroid gland is a remarkable organ with a significant impact on our health and well-being. Its role in regulating metabolism, energy production, and various bodily functions cannot be overstated. Understanding the thyroid gland and its functions is crucial for recognizing the signs of thyroid disorders, seeking appropriate medical care, and taking steps to maintain good thyroid health. In the following sections of this book, we will explore various aspects of thyroid health, including the importance of iodine, the impact of thyroid disorders, and strategies for maintaining thyroid well-being.

The Role of Iodine in Thyroid Gland Health

The thyroid gland, a small but vital organ located in the neck, plays a significant role in regulating numerous bodily functions. Its primary function is to synthesize and release thyroid hormones, thyroxine (T4) and triiodothyronine (T3), which are essential for maintaining metabolism, growth, and overall health. The production of these hormones is highly dependent on the presence of iodine, an essential trace element that plays a crucial role in thyroid function.

In this comprehensive exploration, we will delve into the intricate relationship between iodine and the thyroid gland, understanding how this element is absorbed, utilized, and the profound impact it has on our health. We will also discuss the consequences of iodine deficiency and the importance of maintaining an adequate supply of iodine for optimal thyroid function.

Iodine and Thyroid Hormone Synthesis

The synthesis of thyroid hormones, T4 and T3, begins with iodine. Iodine is an integral component of these hormones, representing approximately 65% of the molecular weight of T4 and 59% of T3. The thyroid gland actively absorbs iodine from the bloodstream to fuel the production of these hormones.

Thyroid follicular cells, where hormone synthesis occurs, have a specialized protein called the sodium-iodide symporter (NIS) on their surface. NIS actively transports iodine from the bloodstream into these cells, where it is then utilized in the production of thyroid hormones.

Once inside the thyroid follicular cells, iodine undergoes a series of chemical reactions. It combines with an amino acid called tyrosine to form both T4 (which contains four iodine atoms) and T3 (which contains three iodine atoms). These hormones are stored in the thyroid follicles until they are needed, at which point they are released into the bloodstream.

Iodine Deficiency: A Silent Epidemic

Iodine is essential for thyroid health, and its deficiency can have profound consequences. When the body lacks sufficient iodine, the thyroid cannot produce an adequate amount of T4 and T3, resulting in a condition known as hypothyroidism. Hypothyroidism is characterized by a slowed metabolism, leading to symptoms like fatigue, weight gain, cold intolerance, and cognitive impairment.

The consequences of iodine deficiency are particularly severe during pregnancy and infancy. Inadequate iodine during these critical periods can lead to developmental issues, intellectual

disabilities, and even cretinism, a severe condition characterized by stunted physical and mental growth.

Iodine deficiency was a widespread problem in the past, leading to initiatives like salt iodization to ensure an adequate iodine supply. However, in some regions and populations, iodine deficiency remains a concern, highlighting the ongoing importance of iodine awareness and supplementation.

Iodine Sources and Recommended Intake

Iodine is not produced by the body, so it must be obtained through diet or supplementation. Seafood, including fish and seaweed, is one of the richest dietary sources of iodine. Other sources include dairy products, eggs, and iodized salt, which is regular table salt fortified with iodine to prevent deficiencies.

The recommended daily intake of iodine varies by age and life stage. For most adults, the recommended daily allowance (RDA) is around 150 micrograms (mcg), but pregnant and breastfeeding women require higher amounts. Adequate iodine intake is crucial to ensure the thyroid can function optimally and maintain overall health.

Iodine Excess and Thyroid Health

While iodine deficiency can lead to hypothyroidism, excessive iodine intake can also negatively affect thyroid health. The condition known as iodine-induced hyperthyroidism or Jod-Basedow phenomenon can occur when an individual consumes excessive iodine, leading to an overproduction of thyroid hormones. This can result in symptoms such as weight loss, anxiety, and heart palpitations.

Iodine excess is often a concern in regions where seaweed is consumed in large quantities, as it contains high levels of iodine. Additionally, some medications and supplements may contain iodine, which, when taken in excess, can disrupt thyroid function.

In conclusion, iodine is an indispensable element for thyroid health and overall well-being. Its essential role in the synthesis of thyroid hormones highlights the intricate relationship between iodine and the thyroid gland. Iodine deficiency can lead to hypothyroidism and a range of associated symptoms, while iodine excess can result in hyperthyroidism.

Maintaining a balanced iodine intake, whether through diet or supplementation, is crucial for supporting optimal thyroid function. Understanding the role of iodine in thyroid health empowers individuals to take charge of their well-being and ensure the proper functioning of this essential organ. In the subsequent sections of this book, we will explore various aspects of iodine supplementation, dietary strategies, and lifestyle choices for maintaining thyroid health.

PART ONE: Iodine Deficiency, A Silent Epidemic

Why Most of Us Are Deficient in Iodine

Iodine is an essential trace element that plays a critical role in maintaining overall health, particularly in regulating the function of the thyroid gland. Despite its importance, a significant portion of the global population, including individuals in developed countries, is deficient in iodine. This deficiency has far-reaching consequences for human health, affecting not only the thyroid but also various other bodily systems and functions. In this comprehensive exploration, we will examine the reasons behind the widespread deficiency of iodine and the implications it has for public health.

1. Dietary Trends and Food Choices

One of the primary reasons for iodine deficiency is the dietary choices made by individuals. Modern dietary trends have shifted away from iodine-rich foods, leading to lower iodine intake. For instance, diets low in seafood, which is a primary dietary source of iodine, can result in insufficient iodine intake. As people increasingly opt for processed and convenience foods over nutrient-dense whole foods, they often miss out on essential nutrients, including iodine.

Moreover, the reduced use of iodized salt in food preparation contributes to the deficiency. Many individuals have switched to non-iodized salt or use less salt altogether due to concerns about sodium intake and blood pressure. This reduction in iodized salt consumption can impact iodine intake significantly, especially in regions where salt is the main dietary source of iodine.

2. Soil Depletion

Iodine levels in food depend on the iodine content in the soil where the crops are grown and the animals are raised. Soil iodine content can vary widely across regions, and some areas have naturally low iodine levels. In such regions, even when individuals consume locally produced foods, they may not receive adequate iodine. Additionally, modern agricultural practices, including the use of fertilizers and irrigation, can further deplete soil iodine content.

3. Vegetarian and Vegan Diets

While plant-based diets can be healthy and environmentally sustainable, they may lack iodine-rich food sources. People following strict vegetarian or vegan diets, which exclude seafood and dairy, can be at a higher risk of iodine deficiency. This is especially concerning when such diets

are not well-planned, and individuals are unaware of the need to obtain iodine from alternative sources.

4. Increased Consumption of Processed Foods

The consumption of processed and convenience foods has risen significantly in recent decades. These foods often contain additives and preservatives that may contain little to no iodine. Additionally, the salt used in processed foods is typically not iodized, further contributing to lower iodine intake in the population.

5. Reduced Fish and Seafood Consumption

Fish and seafood are among the richest sources of dietary iodine. In regions where seafood is not a staple part of the diet, or where economic factors limit access to seafood, iodine intake can be compromised. Preferences for other sources of protein, such as red meat or poultry, can lead to a reduction in fish and seafood consumption.

6. Public Health Measures

Efforts to reduce salt consumption for cardiovascular health have led to recommendations for using less salt in food preparation. While this is a positive step in reducing sodium intake, it can inadvertently reduce iodine intake, as iodized salt is a primary source of dietary iodine in many countries.

7. Misconceptions About Iodine Needs

There are misconceptions about the importance of iodine and the need for iodine supplementation. Some individuals and even healthcare professionals may not fully understand the significance of iodine in thyroid health and overall well-being. As a result, they may not actively seek out or recommend iodine-rich foods or supplements.

8. Regional Disparities

Iodine deficiency is not evenly distributed across the globe. Some regions are more affected than others due to geological and dietary factors. Coastal areas, for instance, often have higher iodine intake due to seafood consumption, while inland regions may face higher rates of deficiency.

9. Government Policies and Regulations

Government policies and regulations play a significant role in addressing iodine deficiency. The implementation of mandatory iodization of salt, for example, has been successful in reducing deficiency in some countries. However, the effectiveness of such policies can vary, and not all nations have adopted iodization programs.

10. The Rise of Specialty Diets

Specialty diets, such as gluten-free diets, which are essential for individuals with celiac disease, can sometimes inadvertently reduce iodine intake. Gluten-free foods often replace wheat with rice and other grains, which may be lower in iodine. This can impact the iodine intake of those with dietary restrictions.

Consequences of Iodine Deficiency

The consequences of iodine deficiency are far-reaching and affect various aspects of health. The most immediate and well-known impact is on the thyroid gland. Iodine deficiency can lead to hypothyroidism, characterized by symptoms like fatigue, weight gain, and cognitive impairment.

In severe cases, it can result in a condition known as endemic cretinism, causing intellectual disabilities and physical deformities.

During pregnancy, iodine deficiency is particularly concerning, as it can lead to developmental issues in the fetus, including intellectual disabilities and stunted growth. Children born to mothers with iodine deficiency are at higher risk of cognitive and motor impairments.

Beyond the thyroid, iodine deficiency can have consequences for cardiovascular health, reproductive health, and the immune system. It may also increase the risk of certain cancers, such as thyroid cancer.

1. Hypothyroidism:

One of the most immediate and well-known consequences of iodine deficiency is hypothyroidism. The thyroid gland relies on iodine to produce its two primary hormones, thyroxine (T4) and triiodothyronine (T3). These hormones are vital for regulating metabolism and ensuring that the body functions optimally.

When iodine levels are insufficient, the thyroid cannot produce enough T4 and T3, leading to an underactive thyroid. Hypothyroidism is characterized by a slowed metabolic rate, which can result in a range of symptoms, including:

- Fatigue: Individuals with hypothyroidism often experience persistent fatigue and low energy levels.

- Weight Gain: Slowed metabolism can lead to unexplained weight gain.

- Cold Intolerance: People with hypothyroidism may feel excessively cold, even in warm environments.

- Cognitive Impairment: Hypothyroidism can affect cognitive function, leading to memory and concentration problems.

- Depression: Changes in hormone levels can contribute to mood disturbances, including depression.

- Dry Skin and Hair: Hypothyroidism can lead to dry, coarse skin and hair.

- Constipation: Slowed digestion can result in chronic constipation.

It's essential to note that hypothyroidism can occur gradually, and many individuals may not recognize the symptoms until they become severe. Untreated hypothyroidism can lead to more severe health issues over time.

2. Endemic Cretinism:

One of the most tragic consequences of iodine deficiency is endemic cretinism. This condition primarily affects infants born to mothers who were iodine deficient during pregnancy. Iodine is essential for the proper development of the fetal brain, and when it's lacking, it can lead to severe intellectual disabilities and physical deformities.

Endemic cretinism is characterized by:

- Profound Intellectual Disabilities: Affected individuals typically have severe cognitive impairments, often unable to communicate or perform basic tasks.

- Physical Deformities: Cretinism can lead to physical abnormalities, including stunted growth, deafness, and muscle weakness.

- Delayed Development: Children with cretinism experience severe developmental delays and may not reach developmental milestones.

Endemic cretinism is particularly prevalent in regions with a high prevalence of iodine deficiency, highlighting the critical importance of iodine for fetal brain development.

3. Developmental Issues:

Iodine deficiency can also lead to developmental issues in children who do not have cretinism. Even mild to moderate iodine deficiency during pregnancy can result in subtle cognitive and developmental impairments in children. These issues may include lower IQ scores, attention problems, and delayed language development.

4. Goiter:

A visible consequence of iodine deficiency is the development of goiter, which is the enlargement of the thyroid gland. The thyroid gland attempts to compensate for the lack of iodine by increasing in size in an effort to produce more hormones. This enlarged thyroid gland can cause a noticeable swelling in the neck, sometimes referred to as a "goiter."

Goiter can lead to physical discomfort, difficulty swallowing, and, in severe cases, it can obstruct the airway, causing breathing difficulties. While goiter itself may not be life-threatening, it is indicative of an underlying iodine deficiency and a malfunctioning thyroid gland.

5. Thyroid Disorders:

Iodine deficiency is a significant risk factor for the development of various thyroid disorders, including autoimmune thyroid diseases such as Hashimoto's thyroiditis and Graves' disease. These conditions can lead to a range of symptoms and complications.

- Hashimoto's Thyroiditis: This is an autoimmune disease where the immune system attacks the thyroid gland. It results in gradual thyroid damage and eventual hypothyroidism.

- Graves' Disease: Graves' disease is another autoimmune disorder that leads to overproduction of thyroid hormones, resulting in hyperthyroidism.

These thyroid disorders can affect individuals of all ages and can have a profound impact on quality of life if not properly managed.

6. Reproductive Health:

Iodine deficiency can also affect reproductive health, particularly in women. It may lead to menstrual irregularities, difficulty conceiving, and an increased risk of pregnancy complications. Pregnant women with iodine deficiency are more likely to have children with developmental issues and intellectual disabilities, as discussed earlier.

7. Cardiovascular Health:

There is evidence to suggest that iodine deficiency can have negative effects on cardiovascular health. While the relationship is complex and not yet fully understood, some studies have linked iodine deficiency to increased risk factors for heart disease, including elevated blood pressure and altered lipid profiles.

8. Immune Function:

Iodine plays a role in immune function, and its deficiency may impact the body's ability to fight off infections. A compromised immune system can make individuals more susceptible to illnesses.

9. Increased Risk of Certain Cancers:

Some research has indicated that iodine deficiency may increase the risk of certain types of cancer, particularly thyroid cancer. While this association is not entirely clear, it underscores the importance of maintaining optimal iodine levels.

10. Mental and Emotional Well-being:

Hypothyroidism resulting from iodine deficiency can have a significant impact on mental and emotional well-being. Depression, anxiety, and cognitive impairments can lead to a diminished quality of life for those affected.

11. Anemia:

Iodine deficiency may also contribute to anemia, as thyroid hormones play a role in red blood cell production.

12. Muscle Weakness and Joint Pain:

Some individuals with iodine deficiency may experience muscle weakness and joint pain, which can affect their mobility and overall quality of life.

Addressing Iodine Deficiency and Preventing Consequences

Preventing the consequences of iodine deficiency requires a multi-faceted approach involving individuals, healthcare professionals, policymakers, and the food industry. Strategies to combat iodine deficiency include:

1. Iodized Salt: Promoting the use of iodized salt in food preparation, especially in regions where iodine deficiency is prevalent, is an effective measure. Public awareness campaigns can educate the public about the benefits of iodized salt.

2. Dietary Education: Encouraging a well-balanced diet that includes iodine-rich foods like seafood, dairy products, and seaweed is essential. Public health campaigns can emphasize the importance of these foods in maintaining iodine levels.

3. Iodine Supplementation: In regions where iodine deficiency is a significant concern, iodine supplementation may be recommended, particularly for vulnerable populations like pregnant women and infants.

4. Public Health Policies: Governments can play a vital role by implementing policies to ensure salt iodization and by monitoring the iodine content of soil in agricultural regions.

5. Healthcare Professional Awareness: Healthcare professionals should be educated about the importance of iodine in thyroid health and overall well-being. This knowledge can lead to better guidance and recommendations for individuals at risk of deficiency.

6. Food Industry Collaboration: The food industry can contribute by incorporating iodized salt into processed foods, ensuring that these products also provide essential iodine.

Conclusion

In conclusion, iodine deficiency is a critical public health concern with a wide range of consequences for human health. The most immediate and well-known impact is on the thyroid, leading to hypothyroidism, goiter, and the development of thyroid disorders. However, the consequences of iodine deficiency extend beyond the thyroid, affecting cognitive development, cardiovascular health, reproductive health, and more.

Addressing iodine deficiency requires a collaborative effort involving individuals, healthcare professionals, policymakers, and the food industry. Public awareness, dietary education, salt iodization, and iodine supplementation can all play essential roles in combating this deficiency and promoting overall health and well-being. Recognizing the consequences of iodine deficiency is a vital step in raising awareness and implementing effective strategies to address this critical public health issue.

PART TWO: The Relationship Between Iodine and Your Thyroid

Iodine Absorption and Utilization in the Body

Iodine is a vital trace element that plays a crucial role in the human body, primarily in the functioning of the thyroid gland. The thyroid gland produces thyroid hormones, thyroxine (T4) and triiodothyronine (T3), which are essential for regulating metabolism and maintaining overall health. To understand the significance of iodine in thyroid health, it's essential to explore how the body absorbs and utilizes iodine. In this comprehensive exploration, we will delve into the intricate processes of iodine absorption, its utilization in the thyroid, and its overall role in maintaining our health and well-being.

Iodine is not naturally produced by the human body, which means it must be obtained from dietary sources. The process of iodine absorption begins in the gastrointestinal system, where iodine is absorbed into the bloodstream and transported to the thyroid gland.

Iodine is primarily found in the diet, with seafood being one of the richest sources. Fish, shellfish, and seaweed are particularly iodine-rich foods. Additionally, dairy products, eggs, and iodized salt are common dietary sources of iodine.

Once iodine-containing foods are ingested, the digestive system plays a vital role in iodine absorption. The iodine in food is primarily in the form of iodide (I-), which is the ion that can be readily absorbed by the body. The stomach and small intestine are key sites for iodine absorption.

In the stomach, iodine in food is primarily in the form of iodate (IO3-) or organic iodine compounds. Stomach acid (hydrochloric acid) plays a role in converting these forms into iodide, which is the bioavailable form for absorption.

Iodide is then transported across the intestinal lining into the bloodstream through a specialized iodide transporter system, which allows iodide to enter the bloodstream and be transported to various tissues in the body.

Iodide is distributed throughout the body via the bloodstream. The concentration of iodide in the blood is relatively low, as the body regulates iodine levels to ensure that it is consistently available for the thyroid gland to produce thyroid hormones.

Iodine Utilization in the Thyroid Gland

The thyroid gland is the primary site of iodine utilization in the body. It actively absorbs iodide from the bloodstream and incorporates it into thyroid hormones. This process is highly regulated to maintain optimal thyroid function and to ensure a steady supply of thyroid hormones.

1. Sodium-Iodide Symporter (NIS):

The sodium-iodide symporter (NIS) is a specialized protein on the surface of thyroid follicular cells. NIS is responsible for actively transporting iodide from the bloodstream into thyroid cells. It uses sodium ions to move iodide against a concentration gradient into the cells.

2. Thyroid Peroxidase (TPO):

Once iodide is inside the thyroid follicular cells, it encounters another crucial enzyme called thyroid peroxidase (TPO). TPO is responsible for the oxidation of iodide to iodine (I_2). This conversion is essential for the subsequent binding of iodine to the amino acid tyrosine, forming the precursors for thyroid hormones.

3. Formation of Thyroid Hormones:

Within the thyroid follicles, iodine combines with tyrosine amino acids to form two primary thyroid hormones: thyroxine (T4) and triiodothyronine (T3). T4 contains four iodine atoms, and T3 contains three. These hormones are then stored in the thyroid gland until they are needed.

4. Release of Thyroid Hormones:

When the body requires thyroid hormones, the thyroid gland releases T4 and T3 into the bloodstream in response to signals from the pituitary gland. T3, being the more biologically active hormone, plays a central role in regulating metabolism and other physiological processes.

Iodine Recycling:

The thyroid gland is highly efficient in its use of iodine. It has a recycling system in place that allows it to reabsorb and reuse iodine from the breakdown of old or excess thyroid hormones. This recycling system is particularly important during periods of iodine deficiency, as it helps the thyroid maintain adequate hormone production even when iodine intake is limited.

Impact of Iodine Deficiency on Thyroid Function:

Iodine deficiency can have a profound impact on thyroid function. When iodine intake is insufficient, the thyroid gland struggles to produce an adequate amount of thyroid hormones.

This can result in hypothyroidism, which is characterized by a slowed metabolic rate and a range of associated symptoms.

Hypothyroidism due to iodine deficiency is a global health concern. Some of the consequences of iodine deficiency on the thyroid and overall health include:

- Fatigue: Low thyroid hormone levels can lead to persistent fatigue.

- Weight Gain: Slowed metabolism can result in unexplained weight gain.

- Cold Intolerance: Individuals with hypothyroidism may feel excessively cold, even in warm environments.

- Cognitive Impairment: Hypothyroidism can affect cognitive function, leading to memory and concentration problems.

- Depression: Changes in hormone levels can contribute to mood disturbances, including depression.

- Dry Skin and Hair: Hypothyroidism can lead to dry, coarse skin and hair.

- Constipation: Slowed digestion can result in chronic constipation.

Iodine Supplementation:

In regions where iodine deficiency is a concern, iodine supplementation can be used as a preventive measure. Iodized salt, for example, contains iodine and is a practical way to ensure an adequate intake. Iodine supplements are also available, but their use should be guided by healthcare professionals, as excessive iodine intake can lead to thyroid dysfunction.

Conclusion: Iodine Absorption and Utilization in the Body

Iodine absorption and utilization in the body are essential processes that underpin thyroid function and overall health. Iodine from dietary sources is absorbed through the gastrointestinal system, converted to iodide, and transported to the thyroid gland. Within the thyroid, iodine is used to synthesize the thyroid hormones T4 and T3, which are critical for regulating metabolism, energy production, and numerous physiological processes.

Understanding the processes of iodine absorption and utilization sheds light on the critical role that iodine plays in maintaining health. Iodine deficiency can lead to hypothyroidism, which has a wide range of consequences for well-being. Recognizing the importance of iodine in thyroid function highlights the significance of a balanced diet, iodized salt, and iodine supplementation in regions where deficiency is a concern. By ensuring adequate iodine intake, individuals can promote optimal thyroid health and overall wellness.

Thyroid Hormone Production

Before diving into thyroid hormone production, it is essential to understand the thyroid gland's anatomy and its role in the endocrine system. The thyroid gland is located in the lower part of the neck, wrapped around the trachea. It consists of two lobes connected by a narrow bridge of tissue known as the isthmus. Each lobe is about the size of a small butterfly wing, and the entire gland weighs roughly 20-60 grams.

The thyroid gland is often referred to as the body's metabolic thermostat because it helps regulate the rate at which cells convert food into energy. It does this by producing thyroid hormones, T4 and T3, which influence the body's metabolic rate and numerous other functions.

Thyroid Hormones: T4 and T3

Thyroid hormones are essential for many physiological processes in the body, including metabolism, growth and development, heart and digestive function, muscle control, brain development, and mood regulation. The two primary thyroid hormones are thyroxine (T4) and triiodothyronine (T3), both of which contain iodine atoms. The difference in their names reflects the number of iodine atoms they contain: T4 has four, while T3 has three.

T4 is the more abundant thyroid hormone, accounting for approximately 80-90% of the total thyroid hormone produced. It is a prohormone, meaning it is relatively inactive on its own. T4 must be converted to T3, the more biologically active form, to have a direct impact on cellular processes. This conversion occurs in various tissues throughout the body, with the primary site being the liver.

T3 is the active thyroid hormone that exerts the most profound influence on metabolic processes. It binds to thyroid hormone receptors in cells, influencing gene expression and regulating energy expenditure. T3 is about ten times more potent than T4, even though it is present in smaller quantities in the bloodstream.

Regulation of Thyroid Hormone Production

The production and release of thyroid hormones are meticulously regulated by a feedback system involving several key players, including the hypothalamus, the pituitary gland, and the thyroid gland itself. This intricate system ensures that thyroid hormone levels remain within a narrow, physiologically optimal range. These organs are :

1. Hypothalamus:

The process begins with the hypothalamus, a region in the brain responsible for maintaining homeostasis in the body. When the hypothalamus senses that thyroid hormone levels are low, it releases thyrotropin-releasing hormone (TRH) into the bloodstream. TRH travels to the next crucial player in the system, the pituitary gland.

2. Pituitary Gland:

The pituitary gland, a pea-sized gland located at the base of the brain, is often referred to as the "master gland" because it controls the release of hormones from other glands. In response to TRH, the pituitary gland releases thyroid-stimulating hormone (TSH) into the bloodstream.

3. Thyroid Gland:

TSH is the key messenger hormone in this system. It travels through the bloodstream and binds to receptors on thyroid follicular cells in the thyroid gland. The binding of TSH to its receptors triggers several essential events within the thyroid gland:

- Uptake of Iodine: TSH stimulates thyroid follicular cells to actively transport iodine from the bloodstream into the cells. Iodine is a critical component of thyroid hormones, and its uptake is the first step in thyroid hormone synthesis.

- Synthesis of Thyroid Hormones: Inside thyroid follicular cells, iodine combines with the amino acid tyrosine to create both T4 and T3. The ratio of T4 to T3 produced depends on the enzymes present within the cells.

- Storage of Thyroid Hormones: Once synthesized, T4 and T3 are stored in the follicular cells within the thyroid gland, waiting for a signal to be released into the bloodstream.

4. Release of Thyroid Hormones:

The final step in thyroid hormone production is the release of T4 and T3 from the thyroid gland into the bloodstream. This release is initiated by a drop in TSH levels, signaling that thyroid hormone levels have risen to an adequate level. The negative feedback loop regulates thyroid hormone production, ensuring that hormone levels remain within the desired range.

T4 to T3 Conversion:

As mentioned earlier, T4 is converted into the more active T3, primarily in peripheral tissues. The conversion of T4 to T3 is essential for thyroid hormones to exert their full effects on various bodily processes. Enzymes known as deiodinases are responsible for this conversion, with the primary site being the liver. While some T3 is produced directly by the thyroid gland, the majority is generated via this peripheral conversion.

Iodine: The Essential Component

Iodine is an indispensable element in the production of thyroid hormones. Without iodine, the thyroid gland would be unable to synthesize T4 and T3. The importance of iodine in thyroid hormone production highlights the critical role of dietary iodine intake.

Iodine is actively transported into thyroid follicular cells from the bloodstream, primarily through a specialized protein known as the sodium-iodide symporter (NIS). This symporter actively pumps iodine against a concentration gradient into the cells, ensuring a constant supply for thyroid hormone synthesis.

Once inside the thyroid follicular cells, iodide is oxidized to iodine by thyroid peroxidase (TPO), an enzyme found within the cells. This oxidation step is crucial for subsequent iodine binding to tyrosine amino acids in the synthesis of T4 and T3.

The thyroid gland is highly efficient in its use of iodine. It has a recycling system in place that allows it to reabsorb and reuse iodine from the breakdown of old or excess thyroid hormones. This recycling system helps maintain an adequate supply of iodine, even when dietary intake is limited.

Thyroid Hormone Binding and Transport:

Thyroid hormones are not freely dissolved in the bloodstream; they are bound to proteins. The two primary thyroid hormone-binding proteins are thyroxine-binding globulin (TBG) and transthyretin. These proteins serve to transport thyroid hormones through the bloodstream and protect them from degradation.

Regulation of Thyroid Hormone Levels:

Thyroid hormone levels in the bloodstream are tightly regulated through the feedback loop involving the hypothalamus, pituitary gland, and thyroid gland. When levels of T4 and T3 are insufficient, the hypothalamus releases TRH, leading to the production and release of TSH by the pituitary gland. This, in turn, stimulates the thyroid gland to produce and release more thyroid

hormones. When levels are adequate, the negative feedback loop inhibits the release of TRH and TSH, preventing overproduction of thyroid hormones.

Effects of Thyroid Hormones on the Body:

Thyroid hormones have far-reaching effects on virtually every cell and tissue in the body. They influence:

- Metabolism: Thyroid hormones regulate the rate at which cells convert food into energy. They increase energy expenditure, heat production, and the breakdown of fats and carbohydrates.

- Heart Function: Thyroid hormones increase heart rate and contractility, playing a role in maintaining normal heart function.

- Temperature Regulation: They help regulate body temperature by controlling heat production.

- Growth and Development: Thyroid hormones are essential for normal growth and development, particularly during childhood and adolescence.

- Muscle Control: They influence muscle contraction and strength.

- Brain Development: Thyroid hormones are critical for brain development, especially in the fetal and early childhood stages.

- Mood and Emotional Well-being: Thyroid hormones can affect mood and emotional states. Hypothyroidism, in particular, is associated with depression and cognitive impairment.

Hyperthyroidism and Hypothyroidism:

Thyroid disorders can result from the overproduction (hyperthyroidism) or underproduction (hypothyroidism) of thyroid hormones. Hyperthyroidism is often characterized by symptoms such as increased heart rate, weight loss, and nervousness, while hypothyroidism presents with fatigue, weight gain, and depression.

Iodine Deficiency and Thyroid Hormone Production:

Iodine deficiency is a global health concern that directly affects the production of thyroid hormones. Without adequate iodine, the thyroid gland cannot synthesize sufficient T4 and T3. This deficiency can lead to hypothyroidism and a range of associated symptoms and complications, including goiter, cognitive impairments, and developmental issues in children.

Conclusion: The Essential Role of Thyroid Hormone Production

In conclusion, the production of thyroid hormones, specifically thyroxine (T4) and triiodothyronine (T3), is a complex and highly regulated process that underpins various physiological functions in the body. The thyroid gland, under the influence of the hypothalamus and pituitary gland, actively synthesizes, stores, and releases these critical hormones.

Thyroid hormones are vital for regulating metabolism, heart function, temperature, growth and development, muscle control, and emotional well-being. Iodine is an essential component in the synthesis of these hormones, highlighting the importance of dietary iodine intake.

Understanding the processes of thyroid hormone production and the factors that influence it is crucial for recognizing the significance of thyroid health. Addressing iodine deficiency through iodized salt, dietary education, and supplementation in at-risk populations is an essential step in ensuring the proper functioning of the thyroid gland and the overall well-being of individuals worldwide.

PART THREE: Iodine Sources and Recommended Intake

Dietary Sources of Iodine

Iodine is an essential trace element that plays a crucial role in the human body. It is a key component of thyroid hormones, which are vital for regulating metabolism, energy production, and overall health. Iodine deficiency can lead to a range of health problems, particularly affecting the thyroid. To understand the importance of dietary sources of iodine, it is essential to explore where iodine comes from, its significance for human health, and strategies for maintaining adequate iodine intake.

The Role of Iodine in the Body

Iodine is primarily known for its critical role in thyroid function. The thyroid gland produces thyroid hormones, thyroxine (T4) and triiodothyronine (T3), which contain iodine atoms. These hormones are crucial for regulating metabolic processes in the body, influencing the rate at which cells convert food into energy. Thyroid hormones also impact body temperature, heart rate, and numerous other physiological functions.

Iodine deficiency can disrupt the synthesis of thyroid hormones, leading to a range of health problems, including hypothyroidism, goiter, and developmental issues in children. The consequences of iodine deficiency underscore the importance of maintaining adequate iodine levels in the body.

Dietary Sources of Iodine

Iodine is not produced by the human body, so it must be obtained from external sources, primarily through the diet. Several dietary sources of iodine provide this essential element to the body. Here are the primary sources of dietary iodine:

1. Seafood:

Seafood, particularly fish and shellfish, is one of the richest natural sources of iodine. Different types of seafood contain varying amounts of iodine, with marine fish typically having higher iodine content than freshwater fish. Some of the iodine-rich seafood options include:

- Cod

- Tuna

- Shrimp

- Haddock

- Sardines

- Mussels

- Salmon

Iodine content can depend on the iodine levels in the water where the seafood is sourced. Seaweed, which grows in iodine-rich marine environments, is exceptionally iodine-rich and is consumed as a delicacy in some cultures.

2. Dairy Products:

Dairy products, including milk, cheese, and yogurt, are good dietary sources of iodine. This is because iodine is used to clean udders and milking equipment in the dairy industry. As a result, iodine residues can be present in dairy products. The iodine content of dairy can also vary depending on the use of iodine-based disinfectants in milking processes.

3. Iodized Salt:

Iodized salt is a common source of dietary iodine in many countries. It is regular table salt to which a small amount of potassium iodide or sodium iodide has been added. Iodized salt is a practical and effective way to ensure adequate iodine intake because salt is a staple in most households and is used in cooking and food preservation. Using iodized salt in food preparation can significantly contribute to iodine intake.

4. Eggs:

Eggs, especially those from hens fed with iodized feed or in regions where the soil is iodine-rich, can be a source of iodine.

5. Seaweed and Seaweed Products:

Seaweed, such as kelp, nori, and dulse, is exceptionally rich in iodine because it absorbs iodine from seawater. In some cultures, seaweed is a common dietary staple, and products like sushi often feature seaweed sheets (nori). However, it's important to note that the iodine content in seaweed can vary widely, and excessive consumption may lead to iodine excess, which can have adverse health effects.

6. Meat:

Meat, such as beef and poultry, can contain varying levels of iodine, depending on the iodine content in animal feed and the environment. In regions where iodine deficiency is not prevalent, meat can contribute to overall iodine intake.

7. Bread and Grains:

In some countries, iodine has been added to bread and grain products as a strategy to address iodine deficiency. This fortification method is particularly effective because these staples are widely consumed.

8. Vegetables and Fruits:

While fruits and vegetables are generally not significant sources of iodine, they may contain small amounts if grown in iodine-rich soil or irrigated with water that contains iodine. The iodine content in plant-based foods tends to be lower and less consistent than in seafood and dairy products.

9. Supplements:

Iodine supplements are available over the counter, and in some cases, healthcare professionals may recommend them to individuals at risk of iodine deficiency, such as pregnant women and those living in regions with known iodine insufficiency. However, the use of iodine supplements should be guided by healthcare professionals, as excessive iodine intake can lead to thyroid dysfunction.

Factors Affecting Iodine Content in Foods

The iodine content of foods can vary widely based on several factors:

Geographical Location:

The iodine content in soil and water can significantly influence the iodine levels in food. Regions near the ocean, with access to iodine-rich marine environments, often have higher iodine content in their local food supply.

Agricultural Practices:

The use of iodine-based fertilizers and feed for livestock can impact the iodine content of crops and animal products.

Food Processing:

Iodine content can change during food processing and cooking. For example, boiling seafood can result in iodine loss as it evaporates into the cooking water.

Iodized Salt Usage:

The use of iodized salt in food preparation is an effective way to ensure adequate iodine intake. In regions where iodine deficiency is a concern, promoting the use of iodized salt is a key public health strategy.

Risks of Iodine Deficiency and Excess

Iodine deficiency can have severe health consequences, primarily affecting the thyroid and overall well-being. Some of the risks associated with iodine deficiency include:

- Hypothyroidism: A slowed metabolic rate, leading to fatigue, weight gain, and cognitive impairment.

- Goiter: An enlargement of the thyroid gland, causing discomfort and potential breathing difficulties.

- Developmental Issues: Iodine deficiency during pregnancy can lead to developmental problems in children, including intellectual disabilities.

- Cognitive Impairments: Even mild to moderate iodine deficiency can lead to cognitive impairments in both children and adults.

- Reproductive Health: Menstrual irregularities, fertility issues, and an increased risk of pregnancy complications.

- Cardiovascular Health: Elevated blood pressure and altered lipid profiles may increase the risk of heart disease.

- Increased Risk of Certain Cancers: Iodine deficiency may be linked to an increased risk of certain cancers, particularly thyroid cancer.

On the other hand, excessive iodine intake can also have adverse effects, leading to hyperthyroidism or thyroid dysfunction. It is essential to maintain iodine intake within recommended levels to avoid both deficiency and excess.

In conclusion, dietary sources of iodine play a vital role in maintaining optimal thyroid function and overall health. Iodine is an essential trace element required for the synthesis of thyroid hormones, which are crucial for regulating metabolism, energy production, and various physiological processes.

Seafood, dairy products, iodized salt, and certain other foods are key sources of dietary iodine. Ensuring adequate iodine intake is crucial to prevent iodine deficiency, which can have far-reaching health consequences, particularly affecting the thyroid and cognitive development. It is equally important to avoid excessive iodine intake, which can lead to thyroid dysfunction.

Promoting awareness of iodine's importance in the diet and advocating for the use of iodized salt in regions at risk of deficiency are critical steps in ensuring that individuals receive the necessary iodine to support their health and well-being. Dietary education and public health efforts can help address iodine deficiency and contribute to better overall health outcomes.

Meeting Your Iodine Needs: A Guide to Adequate Iodine Intake

Iodine is a trace element essential for maintaining optimal thyroid function and overall health. It plays a central role in the synthesis of thyroid hormones, which regulate metabolism, energy production, and numerous physiological processes. Inadequate iodine intake can lead to health problems, particularly affecting the thyroid and cognitive development. To ensure that you meet

your iodine needs, it's essential to understand the importance of iodine, assess your risk of deficiency, and learn how to incorporate iodine-rich foods and iodized salt into your diet.

Iodine is a critical component of thyroid hormones, thyroxine (T4) and triiodothyronine (T3), which are produced by the thyroid gland. These hormones are essential for maintaining various bodily functions, including:

- Metabolism: Thyroid hormones influence the rate at which cells convert food into energy, affecting your overall metabolic rate.

- Temperature Regulation: They help control body temperature and heat production.

- Heart Function: Thyroid hormones impact heart rate and contractility.

- Growth and Development: They play a vital role in growth and development, especially during childhood and adolescence.

- Muscle Control: Thyroid hormones influence muscle contraction and strength.

- Brain Development: They are critical for proper brain development, particularly in fetuses and infants.

- Mood and Emotional Well-being: Thyroid hormones can influence mood and emotional states. Hypothyroidism, in particular, is associated with depression.

To maintain these vital functions and overall health, it is crucial to meet your iodine needs. Insufficient iodine intake can lead to iodine deficiency, which carries various health risks, including hypothyroidism, goiter, cognitive impairments, and developmental problems in children.

Assessing Your Iodine Needs

Meeting your iodine needs begins with understanding your specific requirements. Iodine needs can vary based on age, sex, life stage, and individual factors. Here are some general guidelines for daily iodine intake:

- Infants (0-6 months): 110 micrograms (mcg)

- Infants (7-12 months): 130 mcg

- Children (1-8 years): 90 mcg

- Children (9-13 years): 120 mcg

- Adolescents (14-18 years): 150 mcg

- Adults: 150 mcg

- Pregnant women: 220 mcg

- Breastfeeding women: 290 mcg

These recommended daily allowances (RDAs) provide a baseline for iodine intake, but individual needs can vary based on factors such as activity level, body weight, and health conditions. For example, athletes and individuals with specific medical conditions may require more iodine to support their metabolism and overall health.

Risk Factors for Iodine Deficiency

Determining your risk of iodine deficiency is an essential step in meeting your iodine needs. Several risk factors can increase the likelihood of inadequate iodine intake:

1. Geographical Location: Your location can significantly influence your iodine intake. Regions near the ocean, with access to iodine-rich marine environments, often have higher iodine content in their local food supply. Conversely, landlocked areas or regions with iodine-deficient soil may have lower iodine content in locally sourced foods.

2. Dietary Habits: Your dietary choices can impact iodine intake. If you avoid iodine-rich foods such as seafood, dairy products, and iodized salt, you may be at greater risk of iodine deficiency.

3. Restricted Diets: Vegetarians and vegans, particularly those who avoid iodine-rich foods, may be at risk of iodine deficiency.

4. Pregnancy and Lactation: Pregnant and breastfeeding women have higher iodine requirements to support their own health and the developing fetus or infant.

5. Age: Infants and children have specific iodine requirements for growth and development. Adolescents and young adults may require more iodine to support their active lifestyles.

6. Medical Conditions: Certain medical conditions or treatments, such as radiation therapy or specific medications, can interfere with iodine utilization by the thyroid gland.

7. Use of Non-Iodized Salt: If you primarily use non-iodized salt in your cooking and food preparation, you may not be getting enough iodine from this source.

8. Excessive Iodine Excretion: Some individuals may have a genetic predisposition to excrete iodine more rapidly, which can increase their risk of iodine deficiency even with seemingly adequate intake.

How to Meet Your Iodine Needs

Meeting your iodine needs involves incorporating iodine-rich foods into your diet and, in some cases, using iodized salt. Here are strategies to help you meet your iodine requirements:

1. Include Iodine-Rich Foods:

The most natural way to meet your iodine needs is to include iodine-rich foods in your diet. These foods include:

- Seafood: Fish and shellfish are among the richest sources of iodine. Opt for varieties like cod, tuna, shrimp, haddock, and salmon.

- Dairy Products: Milk, cheese, and yogurt often contain iodine. If you are lactose intolerant or prefer plant-based alternatives, seek out iodine-fortified versions.

- Iodized Salt: When choosing salt for cooking and seasoning, use iodized salt. Iodized salt is a practical and effective way to ensure adequate iodine intake. It is available in most grocery stores.

- Eggs: Eggs can contain iodine, particularly when hens are fed iodine-fortified feed or when produced in regions with iodine-rich soil.

- Seaweed and Seaweed Products: Seaweed, such as kelp, nori, and dulse, is exceptionally rich in iodine. It is a common dietary staple in some cultures.

- Meat: Beef, poultry, and pork can contain varying levels of iodine, depending on factors like animal feed and regional iodine content.

- Bread and Grains: In some regions, iodine has been added to bread and grain products, making them a reliable source of dietary iodine.

2. Be Mindful of Dietary Choices:

Pay attention to your dietary habits and ensure that you incorporate iodine-rich foods regularly. If you have specific dietary preferences, such as vegetarian or vegan diets, consider alternatives that can provide adequate iodine intake. Plant-based iodine sources like iodized plant-based milk can be a suitable option.

3. Use Iodized Salt:

In regions where iodine deficiency is a concern, using iodized salt in food preparation is an effective way to meet your iodine needs. Regularly cooking with iodized salt can significantly contribute to your iodine intake.

4. Educate Yourself:

Stay informed about the iodine content of foods and the potential sources of dietary iodine. By understanding where iodine comes from, you can make informed choices and ensure that you meet your iodine needs.

5. Monitor Your Intake:

If you have specific health concerns, dietary restrictions, or medical conditions that may affect your iodine intake, consult with a healthcare professional or a registered dietitian. They can help you assess your individual iodine needs and develop a tailored dietary plan.

6. Iodine Supplements:

In some cases, healthcare professionals may recommend iodine supplements to individuals at risk of iodine deficiency. These may include pregnant women, breastfeeding women, and those living in regions with known iodine insufficiency. However, the use of iodine supplements should be guided by healthcare professionals to prevent excessive iodine intake.

Risks of Iodine Excess

While it is crucial to meet your iodine needs, it is equally important to avoid excessive iodine intake. Consuming too much iodine can lead to hyperthyroidism or thyroid dysfunction. The tolerable upper intake level (UL) for iodine is approximately 1,100 micrograms (mcg) per day for adults, but individual tolerances can vary.

Excessive iodine intake can occur through the overconsumption of iodine-rich foods or supplements. Therefore, it's vital to strike a balance between meeting your iodine needs and avoiding excessive intake.

A Balanced Approach to Iodine Intake

Meeting your iodine needs is a fundamental aspect of maintaining optimal thyroid function and overall health. Iodine is essential for the production of thyroid hormones, which regulate metabolism, energy production, and various physiological processes. Inadequate iodine intake can lead to iodine deficiency, with associated health risks such as hypothyroidism, goiter, cognitive impairments, and developmental issues in children.

To meet your iodine needs, include iodine-rich foods like seafood, dairy products, and eggs in your diet. Consider using iodized salt in your cooking and food preparation to ensure a reliable source of iodine. Be mindful of your dietary choices and educate yourself about iodine sources to make informed decisions.

If you have specific dietary preferences, restrictions, or health concerns, seek guidance from healthcare professionals or registered dietitians to assess your individual iodine needs. By taking

a balanced and informed approach, you can help maintain optimal thyroid function and overall well-being while avoiding the risks of iodine deficiency and excess.

PART FOUR: The Impact of Iodine Imbalance

Hypothyroidism and Hyperthyroidism: Understanding Thyroid Disorders

Hypothyroidism: An Overview

Hypothyroidism is a condition characterized by an underactive thyroid gland, leading to insufficient production of thyroid hormones. This deficiency can disrupt various bodily functions, resulting in a range of symptoms and health issues.

Causes of Hypothyroidism:

1. Autoimmune Thyroiditis (Hashimoto's Thyroiditis): This is the most common cause of hypothyroidism. It occurs when the body's immune system mistakenly attacks the thyroid gland, impairing its ability to produce hormones.

2. Iodine Deficiency: Inadequate dietary iodine can lead to a reduced capacity for the thyroid gland to synthesize hormones. This condition is more prevalent in regions with low iodine levels in the soil and limited access to iodized salt.

3. Medications: Certain medications, such as lithium and amiodarone, can interfere with thyroid function and lead to hypothyroidism.

4. Surgery or Radiation Therapy: If the thyroid gland is surgically removed or exposed to radiation therapy, it can lead to a deficiency of thyroid hormones.

5. Congenital Hypothyroidism: Some individuals are born with an underactive thyroid gland due to genetic factors.

Symptoms of Hypothyroidism:

The symptoms of hypothyroidism can vary in severity and may include:

- Fatigue and weakness

- Weight gain

- Cold intolerance

- Dry skin

- Constipation

- Hair loss

- Muscle aches and pains

- Joint stiffness

- Depression

- Memory problems

- Slow heart rate

- Menstrual irregularities in women

Diagnosis and Treatment of Hypothyroidism:

Hypothyroidism is typically diagnosed through blood tests measuring thyroid hormone levels. Once diagnosed, treatment usually involves hormone replacement therapy using synthetic thyroid hormones, such as levothyroxine. This medication helps restore thyroid hormone levels to normal and alleviate symptoms.

Hyperthyroidism: An Overview

Hyperthyroidism is the opposite of hypothyroidism; it is a condition characterized by an overactive thyroid gland that produces an excess of thyroid hormones. This excess leads to an acceleration of bodily functions and can result in various symptoms and health concerns.

Causes of Hyperthyroidism:

1. Graves' Disease: This is the most common cause of hyperthyroidism and occurs when the immune system mistakenly stimulates the thyroid gland to produce excess hormones.

2. Toxic Nodular Goiter: Some individuals may develop nodules or lumps in their thyroid gland that produce thyroid hormones independently, without being regulated by the body's feedback mechanisms.

3. Subacute Thyroiditis: This condition can result from inflammation of the thyroid gland, which temporarily releases an excess of hormones into the bloodstream.

4. Excessive Iodine Intake: In rare cases, excessive iodine consumption, often through dietary supplements or certain medications, can lead to hyperthyroidism.

Symptoms of Hyperthyroidism:

The symptoms of hyperthyroidism may include:

- Rapid heartbeat

- Weight loss

- Heat intolerance

- Sweating

- Tremors

- Nervousness and anxiety

- Increased appetite

- Frequent bowel movements

- Muscle weakness

- Sleep disturbances

- Vision problems (in the case of Graves' disease)

Diagnosis and Treatment of Hyperthyroidism:

The diagnosis of hyperthyroidism also involves blood tests to measure thyroid hormone levels. Further tests, such as radioactive iodine uptake and thyroid scans, may be performed to identify the underlying cause. Treatment options for hyperthyroidism include:

- Antithyroid Medications: These medications, such as methimazole or propylthiouracil, can block the production of thyroid hormones by the thyroid gland.

- Radioactive Iodine Therapy: This treatment involves the oral administration of radioactive iodine, which selectively targets and destroys overactive thyroid cells.

- Surgery: Surgical removal of a portion or the entire thyroid gland (thyroidectomy) may be necessary in some cases, particularly if other treatments are ineffective or contraindicated.

The Impact on Patients:

Both hypothyroidism and hyperthyroidism can significantly impact the lives of those affected. Fatigue, mood changes, and weight fluctuations can affect a person's overall well-being and daily functioning. Additionally, these conditions may result in long-term health consequences if left untreated.

Management and Lifestyle Considerations:

Management of thyroid disorders involves a combination of medical treatment and lifestyle considerations. Patients with hypothyroidism typically require life-long medication to replace the missing thyroid hormones. Regular follow-up with healthcare providers is essential to adjust medication doses and monitor thyroid function.

For patients with hyperthyroidism, the choice of treatment may vary based on the underlying cause and individual factors. Antithyroid medications may offer a temporary solution, while radioactive iodine therapy or surgery may provide more lasting results.

In both cases, it is crucial for patients to maintain a balanced and nutritious diet, as well as to manage stress effectively. Stress management techniques, such as mindfulness, relaxation exercises, and therapy, can help alleviate symptoms and improve overall quality of life.

Complications of Untreated Thyroid Disorders:

Untreated thyroid disorders can lead to a range of complications:

Hypothyroidism Complications:

  - Goiter: An enlarged thyroid gland, which can lead to swallowing and breathing difficulties.

  - Cardiovascular Issues: High cholesterol levels, high blood pressure, and an increased risk of heart disease.

  - Mental Health Concerns: Depression, cognitive impairment, and a decreased quality of life.

Hyperthyroidism Complications:

  - Heart Issues: An increased risk of arrhythmias (abnormal heart rhythms), heart disease, and stroke.

  - Osteoporosis: Reduced bone density, leading to an increased risk of fractures.

  - Thyroid Storm: A rare but life-threatening condition characterized by a sudden and severe exacerbation of hyperthyroidism symptoms.

Conclusion: Managing Thyroid Disorders

Hypothyroidism and hyperthyroidism are common thyroid disorders that significantly impact the lives of those affected. While these conditions can pose challenges, timely diagnosis and effective treatment can lead to a significant improvement in patients' well-being.

Understanding the causes, symptoms, and treatment options for these disorders is crucial. Regular medical follow-up and adherence to prescribed treatment regimens, as well as attention to lifestyle factors, play essential roles in managing thyroid disorders.

Moreover, raising awareness about thyroid health and advocating for regular thyroid screening can help in early detection and intervention. By providing comprehensive support and care, healthcare professionals and patients can work together to manage thyroid disorders and achieve a better quality of life.

Autoimmune Thyroid Conditions

Autoimmune thyroid conditions occur when the immune system mistakenly targets the thyroid gland, leading to inflammation and damage. This immune system dysfunction can manifest in two primary ways: as an underactive thyroid (hypothyroidism) or an overactive thyroid (hyperthyroidism). The two most common autoimmune thyroid conditions are Hashimoto's thyroiditis, which leads to hypothyroidism, and Graves' disease, which results in hyperthyroidism.

Hashimoto's Thyroiditis: The Underactive Thyroid Disorder

Hashimoto's thyroiditis is the most common cause of hypothyroidism in the United States and many other parts of the world. It develops when the body's immune system mistakenly targets and attacks the thyroid gland. The exact cause of this autoimmune reaction is not fully understood, but it is believed to involve a combination of genetic and environmental factors. A family history of thyroid disorders and certain viral infections may contribute to the development of Hashimoto's.

Symptoms of Hashimoto's Thyroiditis:

The symptoms of Hashimoto's thyroiditis may include:

- Fatigue

- Weight gain

- Cold intolerance

- Dry skin

- Constipation

- Hair loss

- Muscle aches and weakness

- Depression

- Memory problems

- Slow heart rate

- Menstrual irregularities in women

Diagnosis and Treatment of Hashimoto's Thyroiditis:

Diagnosing Hashimoto's thyroiditis typically involves blood tests to measure thyroid hormone levels and detect the presence of antibodies against the thyroid. These antibodies, such as antithyroid peroxidase (TPO) and antithyroglobulin antibodies, are characteristic of Hashimoto's. Once diagnosed, treatment usually involves hormone replacement therapy using synthetic thyroid hormones, such as levothyroxine. This medication helps restore normal thyroid hormone levels and alleviates the symptoms of hypothyroidism.

Graves' Disease: The Overactive Thyroid Disorder

Graves' disease is the most common cause of hyperthyroidism and results from an autoimmune reaction that stimulates the thyroid gland to produce excessive thyroid hormones. Like Hashimoto's, the exact cause of Graves' disease is not fully understood, but it is believed to involve genetic and environmental factors. Smoking, stress, and viral infections have been associated with an increased risk of Graves' disease.

Symptoms of Graves' Disease:

The symptoms of Graves' disease may include:

- Rapid heartbeat

- Weight loss

- Heat intolerance

- Sweating

- Tremors

- Nervousness and anxiety

- Increased appetite

- Frequent bowel movements

- Muscle weakness

- Sleep disturbances

- Vision problems, such as double vision or eye bulging (in the case of Graves' ophthalmopathy)

Diagnosis and Treatment of Graves' Disease:

Diagnosing Graves' disease typically involves blood tests to measure thyroid hormone levels, as well as the presence of specific antibodies, like thyroid-stimulating immunoglobulins. Additional tests, such as radioactive iodine uptake and thyroid scans, may be performed to identify the underlying cause. Treatment options for Graves' disease include:

- Antithyroid Medications: Medications like methimazole or propylthiouracil can block the production of thyroid hormones by the thyroid gland.

- Radioactive Iodine Therapy: This treatment involves the oral administration of radioactive iodine, which selectively targets and destroys overactive thyroid cells.

- Surgery: Surgical removal of a portion or the entire thyroid gland (thyroidectomy) may be necessary in some cases, especially if other treatments are ineffective or contraindicated.

The Impact on Patients:

Autoimmune thyroid conditions can significantly affect the lives of those who have them. Fatigue, mood changes, and weight fluctuations can disrupt daily functioning and overall well-being. Moreover, these conditions may result in long-term health consequences if left untreated.

Management and Lifestyle Considerations:

Management of autoimmune thyroid conditions typically involves a combination of medical treatment and lifestyle considerations. Patients with Hashimoto's thyroiditis often require lifelong medication to replace the missing thyroid hormones. Regular follow-up with healthcare providers is essential to adjust medication doses and monitor thyroid function.

For patients with Graves' disease, the choice of treatment may vary based on the underlying cause and individual factors. Antithyroid medications may offer a temporary solution, while radioactive iodine therapy or surgery may provide more lasting results.

In both cases, it is crucial for patients to maintain a balanced and nutritious diet, as well as to manage stress effectively. Stress management techniques, such as mindfulness, relaxation exercises, and therapy, can help alleviate symptoms and improve overall quality of life.

Complications of Untreated Autoimmune Thyroid Conditions:

Untreated autoimmune thyroid conditions can lead to a range of complications:

Complications of Untreated Hashimoto's Thyroiditis:

- Goiter: An enlarged thyroid gland, which can lead to swallowing and breathing difficulties.

- Cardiovascular Issues: High cholesterol levels, high blood pressure, and an increased risk of heart disease.

- Mental Health Concerns: Depression, cognitive impairment, and a decreased quality of life.

Complications of Untreated Graves' Disease:

- Heart Issues: An increased risk of arrhythmias (abnormal heart rhythms), heart disease, and stroke.

- Osteoporosis: Reduced bone density, leading to an increased risk of fractures.

- Thyroid Storm: A rare but life-threatening condition characterized by a sudden and severe exacerbation of hyperthyroidism symptoms.

Conclusion: Managing Autoimmune Thyroid Conditions

Autoimmune thyroid conditions, such as Hashimoto's thyroiditis and Graves' disease, significantly impact the lives of those affected. While these conditions can pose challenges, timely diagnosis and effective treatment can lead to a significant improvement in patients' well-being.

Understanding the causes, symptoms, and treatment options for these conditions is crucial. Regular medical follow-up and adherence to prescribed treatment regimens, as well as attention to lifestyle factors, play essential roles in managing autoimmune thyroid conditions.

Moreover, raising awareness about thyroid health and advocating for regular thyroid screening can help in early detection and intervention. By providing comprehensive support and care, healthcare professionals and patients can work together to manage autoimmune thyroid conditions and achieve a better quality of life.

PART FIVE: All You Need To Know About Your Pregnancy And Thyroid

Pregnancy is a remarkable journey filled with excitement and anticipation. It's a time of profound physical and emotional changes, and the well-being of both the mother and the developing fetus is paramount. One aspect of maternal health that often receives significant attention during pregnancy is the thyroid gland, a small but vital organ that plays a crucial role in regulating metabolism and various physiological processes.

Thyroid health is of utmost importance during pregnancy because thyroid hormones are essential for the developing baby's growth and brain development. This comprehensive guide explores everything you need to know about pregnancy and thyroid health, from the significance of the thyroid in pregnancy to common thyroid-related issues, their impact, and strategies to maintain optimal thyroid function during this transformative period.

The Thyroid Gland and Its Role in Pregnancy

Before delving into the specifics of thyroid health during pregnancy, let's understand the thyroid gland's function and its significance for both maternal and fetal well-being.

The thyroid gland is a small, butterfly-shaped organ located in the neck. It produces two primary hormones, thyroxine (T4) and triiodothyronine (T3), both of which contain iodine. These hormones are critical for regulating metabolism, energy production, temperature control, and various bodily functions. During pregnancy, thyroid hormones play a pivotal role in the growth and development of the developing fetus, particularly during the first trimester.

Thyroid Hormones and Pregnancy: A Delicate Balance

Thyroid hormone balance is crucial during pregnancy. A mother's thyroid hormones are not only essential for her own well-being but also for the proper development of the baby's brain and nervous system. It is during the early stages of pregnancy that the baby depends entirely on the mother's thyroid hormones for its thyroid hormone needs.

The demands on the mother's thyroid function increase during pregnancy due to a surge in the production of estrogen and other hormones. As a result, the thyroid gland may need to produce more thyroid hormones to meet these heightened requirements. This balance is precisely why maintaining optimal thyroid function is so critical during pregnancy.

Common Thyroid-Related Issues During Pregnancy

While most pregnant women have no issues with their thyroid function, some may experience thyroid-related complications that can affect both maternal and fetal health. Here are the primary thyroid-related issues that can arise during pregnancy:

1. Hypothyroidism: This is a condition characterized by an underactive thyroid gland, leading to insufficient production of thyroid hormones. If hypothyroidism is not adequately managed during pregnancy, it can lead to developmental issues in the baby, including intellectual and neurological impairments. Additionally, untreated hypothyroidism can result in complications for the mother, such as preeclampsia, anemia, and postpartum hemorrhage.

2. Hyperthyroidism: Hyperthyroidism is the opposite of hypothyroidism; it is characterized by an overactive thyroid gland that produces an excess of thyroid hormones. Uncontrolled hyperthyroidism during pregnancy can lead to premature birth, low birth weight, and even miscarriage. Additionally, maternal complications can include heart problems and preeclampsia.

3. Autoimmune Thyroid Conditions: Autoimmune thyroid conditions, such as Hashimoto's thyroiditis and Graves' disease, can lead to hypothyroidism and hyperthyroidism, respectively. These conditions may require specific management during pregnancy to ensure the mother's and baby's health.

4. Thyroid Nodules and Goiter: Some women may have thyroid nodules or an enlarged thyroid gland (goiter). While most thyroid nodules are benign, some may be cancerous. An evaluation of these nodules may be necessary to determine the appropriate course of action during pregnancy.

5. Thyroid Cancer: Thyroid cancer during pregnancy is relatively rare but can occur. Treatment decisions may involve balancing the need for cancer management with the well-being of the developing fetus.

Screening and Diagnosis During Pregnancy

To ensure maternal and fetal health, it is essential to identify thyroid-related issues promptly during pregnancy. The American Thyroid Association (ATA) recommends universal screening for thyroid dysfunction in pregnant women. This typically involves measuring the levels of thyroid-stimulating hormone (TSH) in the blood. Abnormal TSH levels may indicate a thyroid problem.

Thyroid antibody testing is also conducted in some cases to identify autoimmune thyroid conditions, such as Hashimoto's thyroiditis and Graves' disease. If thyroid dysfunction is detected or suspected, further testing, including the measurement of free T4 and free T3, may be necessary to provide a comprehensive picture of thyroid function.

Thyroid Medication Adjustments During Pregnancy

For pregnant women with pre-existing thyroid conditions or those who develop thyroid dysfunction during pregnancy, proper management is crucial. Thyroid medications, such as levothyroxine for hypothyroidism or antithyroid medications for hyperthyroidism, may need to be adjusted under the guidance of a healthcare provider.

Hypothyroidism: In cases of hypothyroidism, medication doses may need to be increased to maintain adequate thyroid hormone levels during pregnancy. Frequent monitoring and adjustments are often necessary to ensure the health of both the mother and the developing baby.

Hyperthyroidism: Managing hyperthyroidism during pregnancy is complex. Antithyroid medications like methimazole or propylthiouracil are commonly used, but they have potential risks to the developing fetus. The healthcare provider will carefully weigh the risks and benefits and may adjust medication doses as pregnancy progresses.

Effects of Thyroid Medications on Fetal Development

It's important to note that thyroid medications, when appropriately adjusted and monitored, are generally considered safe during pregnancy. Uncontrolled thyroid dysfunction poses a more significant risk to maternal and fetal health than the potential side effects of thyroid medications. The goal is to maintain thyroid hormone levels within the normal range to ensure the best possible outcomes for both the mother and the baby.

Lifestyle and Nutrition Considerations

In addition to thyroid medication management, there are several lifestyle and nutrition considerations that pregnant women can adopt to support their thyroid health:

1. A Balanced Diet: A well-balanced diet that includes a variety of nutrient-rich foods, including iodine and selenium, is essential for overall health and thyroid function. Iodine is particularly important for the production of thyroid hormones. Iodized salt, seafood, dairy products, and eggs

are good dietary sources of iodine. However, it's essential not to overconsume iodine, as excessive intake can lead to thyroid dysfunction.

2. Supplementation: Pregnant women are often advised to take prenatal vitamins, which usually include adequate levels of iodine and other essential nutrients. It's crucial to discuss supplements with a healthcare provider to ensure that they meet individual needs.

3. Stress Management: Pregnancy can be a stressful time, and managing stress is vital for thyroid health. Stress reduction techniques such as meditation, yoga, and mindfulness can help alleviate stress and support overall well-being.

4. Regular Follow-up: Regular check-ups and follow-up appointments with a healthcare provider are essential during pregnancy. These appointments allow for close monitoring of thyroid function and any necessary adjustments to thyroid medications.

The Impact of Thyroid Conditions on Pregnancy Outcomes

The management of thyroid conditions during pregnancy is critical to achieving positive outcomes. When thyroid conditions are well-controlled, the risk of complications for both the mother and the baby is significantly reduced. However, untreated or inadequately managed thyroid issues can result in various complications:

1. Preeclampsia: Uncontrolled hypothyroidism and hyperthyroidism increase the risk of preeclampsia, a condition characterized by high blood pressure and damage to other organs, such as the liver and kidneys.

2. Premature Birth: Hyperthyroidism and uncontrolled thyroid conditions may lead to premature birth, increasing the risk of neonatal complications.

3. Low Birth Weight: Infants born to mothers with unmanaged thyroid conditions may have a lower birth weight, which can be associated with long-term health challenges.

4. Neurological and Developmental Issues: Untreated or poorly managed thyroid conditions, particularly hypothyroidism, can lead to developmental issues in the baby, including intellectual and neurological impairments.

5. Miscarriage: In severe cases of untreated hyperthyroidism, the risk of miscarriage may increase.

Postpartum Thyroid Changes

It's important to note that thyroid health can undergo changes during the postpartum period. Some women may develop postpartum thyroiditis, which can lead to temporary hyperthyroidism followed by hypothyroidism. Postpartum thyroiditis typically occurs within the first year after childbirth and may resolve on its own. However, it requires monitoring and management, especially if it results in hypothyroidism.

Breastfeeding and Thyroid Health

Breastfeeding is encouraged for its numerous health benefits for both the mother and the baby. The thyroid hormones produced by the mother are passed on to the baby through breast milk, playing a crucial role in the infant's growth and development. Therefore, maintaining optimal thyroid function is important for lactating mothers.

Breastfeeding mothers with thyroid conditions, such as hypothyroidism or hyperthyroidism, can safely continue breastfeeding. Medication adjustments may be necessary, but most thyroid medications are compatible with breastfeeding. It's important to consult with a healthcare provider to ensure that any prescribed medications are suitable for breastfeeding.

Conclusion: Thyroid Health and a Healthy Pregnancy

In conclusion, thyroid health is a critical component of a healthy pregnancy. A well-functioning thyroid is essential for both the mother's well-being and the healthy development of the baby. During pregnancy, it's important to undergo proper screening and monitoring for thyroid conditions. If a thyroid issue is identified, appropriate medication management, regular check-ups, and lifestyle considerations can help ensure a healthy pregnancy and a positive outcome for both the mother and the baby.

Pregnancy is a time of anticipation and excitement, and by taking proactive steps to manage thyroid health, expectant mothers can contribute to a smooth and healthy journey into motherhood. For anyone planning to become pregnant or already expecting, discussing thyroid health with a healthcare provider is a critical first step towards a safe and successful pregnancy.

www.ingramcontent.com/pod-product-compliance
Lightning Source LLC
Chambersburg PA
CBHW070737260726

48660CB00007B/2892